THE AGING ANTIDOTES

Your lifelong wellness manual

By

Harry L. Branch

The Aging Antidotes.

Disclaimer.

TABLE OF CONTENTS.

The Aging Antidotes.

Introduction

Scientists have long sought an explanation for aging, and thus far, various ideas have been proposed. Some theories contend that the aging process is natural and that the body is thus preprogrammed to age from birth, while others contend that aging is the consequence of damage accumulating over an extended period of time. According to an analysis of these views, aging is a result of the interplay between genetics, the chemistry of the body's aging chemical processes, physiology, as well as an individual's behavior and attitude.

Though the jury is still out on the utility of antioxidant supplements as disease and age fighters, ingesting more antioxidant-rich fruits and vegetables has well-documented advantages in enhancing health, separate from their antioxidant contents.

The Aging Antidotes.

The American Heart Association and the American Cancer Society do not encourage antioxidant supplements for the general public, but they do suggest a diet with appropriate antioxidant-rich fresh fruits, vegetables, and whole grains. You should also discuss any antioxidant usage with your doctor before you begin. With age comes wisdom...also a lot of aches, pains, and dwindling strength. As you age, your endurance will drop and muscle mass will decline—and that might leave you feeling weary all the time, even with the utilization of natural remedies which can slow down aging. However, a recent investigation may have uncovered a protein that might enable your body to develop blood vessels and muscles like a lot younger individual.

With age comes wisdom...also a lot of aches, pains, and dwindling strength. As you age, your endurance will drop and muscle mass will decline—and that might leave you feeling weary all the time, even with the utilization of natural remedies which can slow down aging. However, a recent investigation may have uncovered a protein that might enable your body to develop blood vessels and muscles like a lot younger individual.

The Aging Antidotes.

The purpose of this book is to educate the thinking of the readers and train them into knowing how aging works, and how to cope with it offering advice on retracing the effects of growing old. If you can believe that you can undoubtedly achieve your desired impression of youthfulness and grasp that becoming old is only a phenomenon of the mind.

The major Antidote to aging relies on how often you can find out time to work it out yourself by doing the needed procedures mentioned in this book.

Every endeavor has been made to make this book as accurate as possible. It was produced to impart information about the fundamental facts of The Aging Antidotes

The eating habit supplies the motivation to follow them. Other notions presented in this book are mine, and others belong to different authors whose books I have read; still, the duty for following them is wholly yours. The content offered is not designed as a diagnosis, cure, or treatment for any sickness or condition. Since adjusting one's diet for the better often causes early cleansing reactions, readers are recommended to educate themselves extensively and receive counsel

The Aging Antidotes.

from a competent health practitioner when necessary. Neither the author nor Publishing has responsibility or duty for any adverse effects that you could face while adjusting your lifestyle.

The Aging Antidotes.

Chapter 1
Aging Research and Science.

Scientists have made enormous strides in their understanding of how to live longer, healthier lives in recent years, which has led to an explosion in the study of longevity.

Their research indicates that aging may actually be a somewhat modifiable process as these researchers continue to learn more about how and why we age. Science-based interventions have the potential to prolong life and slow the aging process. These experts contend that aging may not be unavoidable.

When does aging begin, and what is it?

As cellular damage builds up with age, function gradually declines.

Aging, in a broader sense, is the result of the physiological changes that take place over the course of our lifetimes. While some of these changes appear to be unimportant (such as hair graying and wrinkles), others have a more significant effect, affecting things like mobility, bone strength, and disease susceptibility.

The Aging Antidotes.

The fourth decade of life, or between the ages of 30-39 years, is thought to be when the complex, non-linear process of aging is thought to start.

However, everyone ages differently. While some people continue to function mentally and physically well into their later years, others start to show signs of aging as early as their mid-20s. The rate of aging is significantly influenced by behavioral and psychological factors, such as diet, physical activity, smoking status, stress levels, sleep patterns, and social connections, in addition to genetics and biology, which play a significant role.

Age-Related Theories

Scientists have speculated for years about the precise mechanisms underlying the process to understand its cause, and effect, and what prevents it given the inherent complexity of aging. Over 300 theories were once put forth to explain the phenomenon. Later pages of this book will highlight some of the theories.

Two major categories of aging have emerged as a result of advances in research aimed at understanding the process: Programmed theories of aging and Damage theories of aging.

Programmed Theory Of Aging.

The central tenet of programmed theories is that aging is a biological necessity. Cells are designed to age and purposefully lose function over time. In other words, a cell's life span is limited.

Genetic theory: In this theory, turning certain genes "on" and "off" is what causes aging.

Endocrine theory: This theory relates hormone levels to the rate of aging. Hormone levels that regulate functions like blood sugar regulation decline with age and lead to cellular process dysregulation.

The immune system is programmed to peak during adolescence and decline over time, leading to an increased susceptibility to illness and disease, according to the immunological theory.

Aging Damage Theory.

Aging is not seen as a natural process, but rather as the accumulation of environmental damage, according to damage theories of aging.

The Aging Antidotes.

This hypothesis holds that the primary causes of aging are wear and tear.

Wear and tear theory: According to this theory, tissues and cells are not very healthy.

Aging Types, Causes, and Prevention, Aging Healthier.

We all age, but we don't know much about it. It's simple to list all the changes that occur as we get older, such as memory loss, wrinkles, and lean muscle loss, but no one really knows what aging is, why it occurs, or whether we can slow it down or stop it.

Age: What Is It?

Aging is "that which occurs to our bodies over time," so think of it that way. This definition covers the various changes that the human body experiences as it ages (as opposed to the signs of aging, such as gray hair and wrinkles).

The body can age in some cases, like when a child goes through puberty and experiences growth spurts. Aging can also be cumulative, as in the case of skin aging brought on by too much sun exposure.

The Aging Antidotes.

In the end, aging is a result of both physiological changes in our bodies and environmental factors. While the former is frequently out of our control, some environmental factors can be changed and may have an impact on how quickly we age.

How Quickly Does Your Body Age?

Aging styles

When we delve deeper into the aging process, we find theories that explain how and why our bodies age on various levels.

Aging of Cells

Before the genetic material can no longer be accurately copied, a cell can replicate about 50 times. Cellular senescence, which occurs when replication fails, is the process by which a cell loses its ability to function. The characteristic of cellular aging, which translates to biological aging, is the accumulation of senescent cells.

The more free radicals and environmental factors harm cells, the more cells must replicate, and the faster cellular senescence sets in.

The Aging Antidotes.

Hormonal Aging.

Hormones play a significant role in aging, particularly during childhood when they support the development of secondary male or female characteristics and aid in bone and muscle growth. Numerous hormones will gradually start to produce less of themselves, which will modify the skin (causing wrinkles and a lack of suppleness) as well as muscle tone, bone density, and sexual desire.

Males and females have different levels of sex hormones, which affects how they age.

Accumulated Injury

Wear and tear, often known as cumulative damage-induced aging, refers to the external forces that can accumulate over time. The body might suffer effects from exposure to chemicals, UV radiation, unhealthy meals, and pollution, to name a few.

These outside elements have the potential to harm cells' DNA directly over time (in part by exposing them to excessive or persistent inflammation). The body's capacity to restore itself may be compromised by Cumulative damage, hastening the aging process.

What Amount of Skin Aging Does Sunscreen Slow?

Biological Aging

Your cells are continually converting food into energy as you go about your day, which creates byproducts, some of which can be damaging to the body. Despite being necessary, the process of metabolization can gradually harm cells, a condition known as metabolic aging.

Some specialists think that methods like calorie restriction and metabolic slowdown may help humans age more slowly. Blood Iron Levels May Play a Major Role in Healthy Aging

Growing Older.

Growing older is inevitable, despite our age-obsessed culture's obsession with "slowing down aging" and extending life. Your body will alter in important ways regardless of what you do.

For instance, by the time a person reaches the age of 20, their lung tissues will start to lose their flexibility, their

The Aging Antidotes.

rib cage muscles will start to weaken, and their general lung function will start to steadily decline.

Similarly, as we become older, the production of digestive enzymes will start to slow down, which has an impact on how nutrients are absorbed by the body and the kinds of food we can easily digest.

As we age, blood vessels become less flexible. Atherosclerosis can result from the loss of elasticity combined with the buildup of fatty deposits in sedentary individuals who consume poor diets "hardening of the arteries"

Vaginal secretions will drop as a woman approaches menopause, and the loss of estrogen will cause the sexual tissues to begin to atrophy. As testosterone levels drop in men, lean muscle will deteriorate and sperm production will decline.

How to Delay Aging.

You cannot stop aging. Having said that, there are a number of things you can do to reduce the environmental influences on aging:

Eat Sensibly.

The Aging Antidotes.

The body suffers damage from extra sugar, salt, and saturated fat, which raises the risk of hypertension, diabetes, and heart disease. Increase your consumption of fruits, vegetables, nutritious grains, low-fat dairy, lean meat, and fish to prevent these aging-related issues.

Examine Labels.

If you purchase packaged foods for convenience, read the labels to make sure you keep your daily sodium consumption below 1,500 milligrams (mg), your daily sugar intake below 25, and your daily intake of saturated fats below 10% of your daily caloric intake.

Give Up Smoking.

Quitting smoking lowers your risk of cancer significantly while enhancing circulation and blood pressure. There are effective cessation tools that can help, even if it frequently takes repeated efforts to finally break the habit.

Exercise.

The majority of folks do not exercise enough to maintain excellent health (roughly 30 minutes of moderate to strenuous exercise 5 days per week).

The Aging Antidotes.

However, compared to not exercising, 15 minutes of moderate movement every day can increase longevity.

Socialize.

Socialization keeps us mentally active and may also have an impact on our longevity. 11 Keep up healthy, positive ties with other people. Keep in touch with the individuals you care about, and make an effort to meet new people.

Get Enough Rest.

Shorter lifespans and lower health are associated with long-term sleep deprivation. You may feel better and live longer if you practice better sleep hygiene and obtain 7 to 8 hours of sleep each night.

Reduce Stress.

Chronic stress and anxiety can be damaging to your body as they trigger the release of an inflammatory stress hormone called cortisol. Learning to control stress with relaxation techniques and mind-body therapies may help alleviate the indirect inflammatory pressure placed on cells. Our bodies will not live forever as they also have vital parts that wear out with continued use.

Rate of Living Theory: Based on this theory, the rate of an organism's metabolism determines lifespan, with a faster metabolism resulting in a shorter lifespan.

Cross-linking theory: According to this theory, aging occurs as cross-linked proteins accumulate and damage cells and tissues.

Free-Radical Theory:This theory proposes that aging is caused by environmental free-radical exposure, which damages DNA, proteins, and lipids. Environmental exposures to cigarette smoke, pollution, and ultraviolet rays contribute to free radical production.

Genome instability theory: This theory states that aging results from damaged DNA, particularly mitochondrial DNA, that the body has been unable to repair. Over time, this damaged DNA accumulates and further hinders the DNA repair process. We Don't Have To Attribute aging to a loss of Information as cells become damaged they lose the information encoding their identity. As damage accumulates, more cells lose their

The Aging Antidotes.

identity, and tissue and organ function begin to decline and result in aging.

Can you slow aging?

As research evolves, aging experts are reframing the aging process. Rather than just a set of innate biological processes that result in irreversible molecular and cellular changes, aging is a complex interaction between genetics and lifestyle. While genes are hereditary, research shows that individuals have the power to extend their lifespan by altering key lifestyle aspects like diet, exercise, stress, and sleep.

Science-Backed Anti-Aging Habits.

While longevity may be the ultimate goal, these interventions not only focus on extending lifespan but extending healthspan—the number of years we live in good health—as well.

Eat broccoli sprouts: Broccoli sprouts are packed with sulforaphane, a powerful anti-aging compound. Sulforaphane activates pathways in the body that suppress inflammation, activate detoxification, and promote antioxidant action.

The Aging Antidotes.

Get Quality Sleep—but not too much: The body's repair mechanisms occur while we sleep. One study examining the sleep habits of 1.3 million individuals found that those who slept between six to nine hours per night had the lowest risk of all-cause mortality compared to those who slept for less than six or more than nine hours per night.

Reduce Red Meat Intake: Red and processed meat intake are associated with a greater risk of all-cause mortality and mortality from cardiovascular disease, the number one cause of death in the United States. According to one study, swapping red meat for plant-based protein sources like beans or tofu is associated with a 13% lower risk of mortality in men and a 15% lower risk of mortality in women.

Consider Intermittent Fasting: Intermittent fasting contributes to longevity by eliciting the adaptive stress response within the body - a positive type of physiological stress. Adaptive stress activates different pathways in the body that help to increase the production of antioxidants, stimulate DNA repair, decrease inflammation, and clear out dead and damaged cells.

The Aging Antidotes.

Keep stress levels in check: It is well established that high-stress levels negatively impact almost every aspect of health, including longevity. Research shows that those who can manage stress and experience positive emotions like happiness and joy live longer, healthier lives.

Key Takeaways

Aging is a decrease in functional capacity over time due to accumulated cellular damage.

There is not one singular explanation as to why we age. Rather, aging is the result of complex interactions between our genetics and our environment.

There are two main categories of aging: programmed theories and damage theories.

Based on the most recent scientific advances, researchers believe that the aging process can be slowed down.

Eating a well-balanced diet, getting enough sleep, and managing stress levels are three key interventions that longevity experts agree on.

The Aging Antidotes.

Chapter 2
The Ageist Philosophy

In reality, death or the termination of reproduction (or at least of reproductive usefulness) determines how natural selection works and influences the death rate. Because I believe an old tree in the forest has a greater anticipation of the future than a young one, I don't think the father oak should profit from the kid unless he can do so while losing much less than the offspring receives. The reproductive value at various ages must be used to gauge how much parental care costs. If all ages were equally desirable for reproduction , a specie would prefer to favor its kid up to the point at which the offspring gains double the benefit that the parent loses, but not beyond. In actuality, small children are frequently given far less value and should only receive less expensive care. But if crocodiles could recognize their fully developed offspring, I imagine they would cooperate with them for both their individual and collective good, so long as the loss of one did not outweigh the gain of the other by more than two to one. As a result, the family is the foundation of society.

The Aging Antidotes.

Since it was found that caloric restriction may slow down the aging process and lengthen animal lifespans, it has been close to a century. The same traits are also seen in other research models species such as fish, worms, flies, and yeast.

There is an evolutionary history between diet, environmental factors, and aging, claims Kristopher Burkewitz, Ph.D., associate professor of cell and developmental biology at Vanderbilt. And it all makes sense. When resources are few, it is not a good investment to put energy into growing and producing offspring. Instead, reprogramming takes place on a variety of biological levels to direct energy toward taking care of things and enduring challenging periods. Two years is the maximum duration, however, that is not long enough to understand long-term impacts.

We're talking about decades-long research to genuinely determine that nutritional interventions are effective in individuals, says Rafael Arrojo e Drigo, Ph.D., associate professor of Molecular Physiology and Biophysics.

The Aging Antidotes.

He adds that other factors, including genetics, sex, environment, and lifestyle factors, need to be included in the investigations.

"How do you know it's functioning? What types of tests can you perform on a person to see whether they are changing in terms of biological age as opposed to chronological age?

At this time, there isn't enough data to recommend a particular fasting or calorie-restricted diet. Follow the tried-and-true advice to eat balanced meals of nutritious foods, exercise often, participate in social activities, refrain from smoking, drink alcohol in moderation or not at all, and get a good night's sleep, advise researchers.

The Aging Antidotes.

Chapter 3
Dietary Supplements as Antidote For Aging.

You may use dietary supplements to increase the nutrients in your diet or to reduce your chance of developing conditions like osteoporosis or arthritis. Dietary supplements are available as tablets, capsules, powders, gel caps, liquids, extracts, and pills. They might have herbs or other plants, enzymes, fiber, vitamins, minerals, or amino acids. The components of dietary supplements are occasionally added to meals and beverages. Purchasing nutritional supplements does not need a prescription from a physician.

Will a dietary supplement help me?

The best approach to receiving the nutrients you require is to eat a variety of healthful meals. However, some individuals could not consume enough vitamins and minerals in a given day. When that occurs, their doctors can advise a nutritional supplement to make up for the nutrients they are lacking.

The Aging Antidotes.

When considering utilizing dietary supplements:

Do as much research as you can on any dietary supplements you are considering using. Speak to your physician, pharmacist, or licensed dietician. It is possible that a supplement won't work for you even though it helped your neighbor. Be careful of the information's source when reading fact sheets or browsing websites. Could the author or group make money from the sale of a specific supplement? Learn more about selecting trustworthy sources for health information.

Remember, Something is not necessarily safe or healthy for you just because it is described as "natural." It could have negative effects. It might either weaken or strengthen a medication that your doctor recommended for you. If you have specific medical issues, it can potentially hurt you.

Tell your physician:

Consult your doctor before beginning to take a dietary supplement to address any medical issue. Without first seeing your doctor, never try to diagnose or treat any medical issue with a supplement. Learn how dietary supplements and drugs may interact. Visit the National Center for Complementary and Integrative Health for further details.

Buy sensibly.

A doctor's, dietitian's, or pharmacist's recommended brands should be used. Buy no dietary supplements that include substances you don't require. Contrary to popular belief, taking too many supplements or those with a very high concentration of a vitamin can be detrimental. Spending money on unnecessary supplements is feasible.

Look into science.

Make sure every assertion made regarding a dietary supplement is supported by research. The United States Pharmacopeia (USP) certified mark should be visible. The identification, excellence, potency, and purity of supplements are all verified by USP. MedlinePlus has information on various dietary supplements, but it's crucial to remember that the majority of them have scant evidence supporting their efficacy. Anything that seems too wonderful to be true probably is.

The Aging Antidotes.

Be a wise shopper.

Some dietary supplement advertising in periodicals, online, or on TV claims that certain items may improve your health, stave off illness, or even lengthen your life. It's crucial to understand that frequently, there is little to no evidence to back up these assertions.

vitamins for older folks' diets

Compared to younger folks, those over 50 may require more vitamins and minerals. If you don't receive enough of these, your doctor or a nutritionist can advise you if you need to adjust your diet or take a vitamin or mineral supplement:

Calcium: Calcium helps maintain bones healthy at all ages by collaborating with vitamin D. Fractures can result from bone loss in both elderly men and women. Calcium may be found in milk and milk products (low-fat or fat-free is preferable), canned fish with soft bones, kale, and foods with additional calcium, such as breakfast cereals.

The Aging Antidotes.

Vitamin D: The majority of Americans don't get the necessary quantity of vitamin D. Discuss with your doctor if you should use a vitamin D supplement or increase your intake of fatty fish, vitamin D-fortified cereals, and milk and milk products.

Vitamin B6: Red blood cells require this vitamin to develop. Potatoes, bananas, chicken breasts, and fortified cereals all contain it.

Vitamin B12: This supports the functioning of your neurons and red blood cells. While older persons require the same amount of vitamin B12 as normal adults, some older adults have problems absorbing the nutrient. Your doctor could advise you to consume foods like fortified cereals with this vitamin added or take a B12 supplement if you have this issue. Due to the fact that animal products are the only natural dietary sources of vitamin B12, strict vegetarians and vegans are more likely to have vitamin B12 insufficiency. Consult your doctor to determine if taking a B12 supplement is appropriate for you.

recommendations for vitamins and minerals for individuals over 50.

The Aging Antidotes.

The recommended daily allowances for each vitamin and mineral for men and women of various ages are provided in the Dietary Guidelines for Americans, 2020–2025. For instance:

2.4 mcg (micrograms) of vitamin B12 daily. Your healthcare practitioner can offer you information on whether you need a different version of the medication if you are taking it for acid reflux.

Women over 50 years old require 1,200 mg (milligrams) of calcium daily. Men require 1,200 mg beyond the age of 70 and 1,000 mg between the ages of 51 and 50, but no more than 2,000 mg each day.

For adults over 70 and those between the ages of 51 and 70, the recommended daily intake of vitamin D is 800 IU (international units), but no more than 4,000 IU.

Men need 1.7 mg of vitamin B6 daily, while women need 1.5 mg.

A vitamin or mineral taken in excess might occasionally be detrimental. Your daily vitamins and minerals should primarily—if not entirely—come from food. Think

The Aging Antidotes.

about how much of each nutrient you get from food and drink, as well as from any supplements you take when determining if you need more of a certain vitamin or mineral. To find out whether you need to supplement your diet, consult a doctor or nutritionist.

How do antioxidants work?

Antioxidants may be mentioned in the news. These are components of food that are naturally occurring and may offer some disease defense. You should make sure to incorporate the following typical antioxidants in your diet:

Dark green or dark orange fruits and vegetables contain beta-carotene. Selenium is present in cereals, fish, pork, and liver.

Citrus fruits, peppers, tomatoes, and berries all contain vitaminC.

Wheat germ, almonds, sesame seeds, canola, olive, and peanut oils all contain vitamin E.

According to current studies, using antioxidant supplements at high levels won't stop chronic illnesses like diabetes or heart disease. Several studies have indicated that consuming some antioxidants at significant levels may be detrimental. It is essential to consult your doctor before using a dietary supplement, as before.

Older adults and herbal supplements.

Dietary supplements that derive from plants are known as herbal supplements. Whether they come in the form of a capsule, tablet, powder, or liquid, these supplements are consumed orally.

Some of these include ginkgo Biloba, ginseng, echinacea, and black cohosh, which you may have heard of. Although it's still too early to tell if herbal supplements are both safe and effective,

researchers are investigating utilizing them to cure or prevent various health issues. Previous research on several herbal supplements failed to find any advantages.

It's crucial to understand that just because a supplement is natural or derived from plants, it doesn't automatically imply that it is secure.

The Aging Antidotes.

Are nutritional supplements secured?

The Food and Drug Administration (FDA) of the United States examines prescription medications, such as antibiotics and blood pressure medications, to ensure that they are effective and safe. The same is true for over-the-counter medications like cold and pain relievers. Dietary supplements, on the other hand, are not under the control of the FDA and are not subject to its approval for safety or efficacy prior to being made available to the general public.

The FDA is not obliged to be informed about the safety of these items before they are sold by firms, and the federal government does not routinely analyze the ingredients in dietary supplements. A dietary supplement may not be safe, perform what it claims to do, or contain what it claims to contain simply because it is on a shop shelf.

The FDA will publish warnings about a supplement if it learns of complaints of potential issues with it. Supplements that are deemed hazardous may potentially be taken off the market by the FDA.

The Aging Antidotes.

The Federal Trade Commission looks into complaints about advertisements that may exaggerate the benefits of dietary supplements. A few private organizations, like the Natural Products Association, ConsumerLab.com, NSF International, and the U.S. Pharmacopeia, have their own "seals of approval" for dietary supplements. Products must adhere to good manufacturing practices in order to receive this certification, include just the contents mentioned on the label, and not contain dangerous amounts of unwanted elements, such as lead. Whether you use dietary supplements or not, maintaining a healthy lifestyle is always crucial. Try maintaining a nutritious diet, engaging in regular exercise, thinking critically, quitting smoking, and visiting your doctor frequently.

The Aging Antidotes.

Chapter 4
How Age Works

Organs, tissues, and cells change as we age.

As you become older, every critical organ starts to perform less and less. All of the body's cells, tissues, and organs experience aging-related changes, which have an impact on how each bodily system functions.

Cells make up the tissue of living things. Cells come in a wide variety of varieties, yet they always share the same fundamental structure. Layers of identical cells that carry out a certain role make up tissues. Organs are constructed from a variety of tissues.

Four fundamental forms of tissue exist:

Other tissues are held together and supported by connective tissue. This comprises the tissues that support and shape the skin and internal organs, as well as the bone, blood, and lymph tissues. For both the surface and deeper layers of the body, epithelial tissue serves as a covering. Epithelial tissue makes up the skin and the lining of internal organs like the gastrointestinal

The Aging Antidotes.

tract. Three different tissue types make up muscle tissue:

muscles that are strained, such as those that move the skeleton (also called voluntary muscle)

Smooth muscles, sometimes known as involuntary muscles, are those found in the female uterus, the stomach, and other internal organs.

Mostly comprised of cardiac muscle, the heart wall (also an involuntary muscle)

Neurons, the building blocks of nerve tissue, are utilized to transmit signals to and from different sections of the body. Nerve tissue makes up the brain, spinal cord, and peripheral nerves.

AGES AND CHANGES

Tissues are composed primarily of cells. Aging causes alterations in all cells. They enlarge and lose their capacity for division and multiplication. In addition to other modifications, the cell's inside now contains more colors and fatty compounds (lipids). Numerous cells either stop functioning correctly or start to do so.

The Aging Antidotes.

Waste materials accumulate in tissue as we age. Many tissues accumulate lipofuscin, a fatty brown pigment, along with other fatty compounds.

The stiffness of connective tissue increases with age. The airways, blood arteries, and organs become stiffer as a result. Because cell membranes deteriorate, it is harder for many tissues to absorb nutrients and oxygen and to expel wastes like carbon dioxide.

Numerous tissues lose bulk. We refer to this process as atrophy. Some tissues grow more stiff or lumpy (nodular). Your organs alter as you age due to cell and tissue changes. Organs that are aging gradually stop working. Because you rarely need to use your organs to their full potential, the majority of individuals do not immediately realize this loss.

Organs are capable of functioning in excess of what is normally required. For instance, a 20-year- old may pump around 10 times as much blood than is actually required to maintain life in the body. After the age of 30, this reserve decreases annually on average by 1%. The heart, lungs, and kidneys see the largest alterations in organ reserve. The quantity of reserve that is lost

The Aging Antidotes.

varies across individuals and between various organs within a single individual.

These changes take a while to manifest and happen gradually. An organ may not be able to enhance function when exercised harder than normal. When the body is working harder than normal, issues like sudden heart failure or other issues might arise. The following are examples of factors (or body stresses) that increase workload:

Illness\Medicines.

significant changes in life increased physical demands placed on the body suddenly, such as those caused by a shift in exercise or exposure to an altitude.

It is also more difficult to return the body to homeostasis when the reserve is lost. The liver and kidneys eliminate drugs from the body more slowly than other organs. Side effects become more frequent and medication dosages may need to be decreased. Rarely do diseases completely heal, which causes increased levels of impairment.

It is simple to confuse a drug reaction for sickness since the side effects of medication can resemble the signs of numerous ailments. Some medications have completely different negative effects on older patients compared to younger patients.

AGING THEORY

Nobody is aware of how or why people change as they age. According to some hypotheses, aging is brought on by damage from UV radiation over time, physical wear and tear, or metabolic waste products. According to some ideas, aging is a genetically set process.

There is no one process that can account for all of the aging changes. Aging is a complicated process that affects various persons and even different organs differently. The majority of gerontologists (scientists who research aging) believe that a variety of factors throughout one's life combine to cause aging. These factors include inheritance, environment, culture, food, physical activity, prior medical conditions, and many others.

Each individual matures at a different rate, in contrast to the changes associated with puberty, which are predicted to occur within a few years. Some systems start to age as early as 30 years old. Other forms of aging do not appear until much later in life. Even if there are some changes that come with becoming older, they happen at various rates and to varying degrees. You cannot precisely foresee how you will age.

TERMS TO DEFINE DIFFERENT KINDS OF CELL CHANGES.

Atrophy: Cells get smaller. The entire organ atrophies if enough of the cells experience a size decline. This is frequently a typical aging alteration that can affect any tissue. The heart, brain, sex organs, and skeletal muscle are where it most frequently occurs (such as the breasts and ovaries). With modest stress, bones grow thinner and more brittle.

Although the exact origin of atrophy is uncertain, some factors include decreased effort, decreased blood flow to the area, decreased nourishment of the cells, and diminished stimulation from hormones or nerves.

Cells expand due to hypertrophy. Instead of an increase in cell fluid, this is brought on by an increase in proteins in the cell membrane and other cell components.

To compensate for the loss of cell mass caused by certain cells atrophying, other cells may hypertrophy.

The Aging Antidotes.

Hyperplasia: An increase in cell count. The rate of cell division is increasing.

Usually, hyperplasia takes place to make up for cell loss. It enables the skin, gut lining, liver, and bone marrow to regenerate among other organs and tissues. The liver excels in regeneration in particular. Within two weeks following damage, it may replace up to 70% of its structural integrity.

Bone, cartilage, and smooth muscle are examples of tissues that have a restricted capacity to regenerate (such as the muscles around the intestines). The nerves, skeletal muscle, heart muscle, and the lens of the eye are tissues that seldom or never regenerate. These tissues are replaced by scar tissue after injury.

Dysplasia: An abnormality in the size, shape, or arrangement of mature cells. Additionally known as atypical hyperplasia.

The cervix's cells and the lining of the respiratory system frequently exhibit dysplasia.

Neoplasia: The development of tumors, whether malignant (cancerous) or benign (benign).

The Aging Antidotes.

Neoplastic cells frequently divide rapidly. They could have odd forms and strange functionalities.

Your body will change as you get older, including the following changes:

hormone synthesis

Immunity.

The skin

Sleep

Bones, muscles, and joints

The breasts

The face

The female reproductive system

The heart and blood vessels

The kidneys

The lungs

The male reproductive system

The nervous system.

The Aging Antidotes.

Chapter 5
Physical Exercises That Delay Aging.

To investigate if exercise may slow down aging, researchers set out to evaluate the health of older persons who had been physically active for most of their adult life.

125 amateur cyclists between the ages of 55 and 79 were selected for the study; 84 of them were men and 41 were women. The required cycling distances for the men and women were 100 km for the men and 60 km for the ladies. The study eliminated those who smoked, drank excessively, had high blood pressure, or had any other medical issues.

The participants performed a battery of lab tests, and their results were contrasted with those of a group of people who don't engage in regular physical exercise. This cohort included 55 healthy young adults between the ages of 20 and 36 and 75 healthy individuals between the ages of 57 and 80.

Numerous activities can slow down and limit aging quickly in both men and women; some of these activities may be impacted as aging progresses or as one approaches advanced age. These are what they are:

Activities and routines for the body(Exercises and physical workouts).

Having enough sleep and rest(Sleeping and Resting Enough).

Affection and sex(Touch And Sex).

Activities And Routines For The Body (Exercises and physical workouts.):

 A study found that those who exercise consistently do not lose strength or muscular mass. The bikers' body fat, cholesterol, and testosterone levels did not rise as they aged, and the men's levels of the hormone also stayed high, suggesting that they may have mostly avoided male menopause.

Surprisingly, the study also showed that the advantages of exercise go beyond muscle since the riders' immune systems appeared to have remained youthful.

From the age of 20, the thymus, an organ that produces T cells, a kind of immune cell, begins to decrease. However, in this study, the thymuses of the bikers were producing an equal number of T cells as those of a young individual.

The findings coincide with data showing that more than half of those over 65 have at least two ailments and that fewer than half of individuals over 65 exercise enough to be healthy. "Hippocrates in 400 BC declared that exercise is man's finest medicine, but his message has been lost over time and we are an increasingly sedentary culture," said Professor Janet Lord, Director of the Institute of Inflammation and Aging at the University of Birmingham. However, our data disprove the notion that growing older inevitably makes us more feeble.

Strong evidence from research suggests that encouraging individuals to commit to regular exercise throughout their lives is a workable solution to the issue of our longer lifespans without improving our health."We hope these results avert the danger that, as a culture, we accept that old age and sickness are typical bedfellows and that the third age of man is something to be endured and not enjoyed," said Dr. Niharika Arora Duggal, also of the University of Birmingham.

The Aging Antidotes.

The results highlight the reality that the bikers are healthy because they have been exercising for such a significant period of their life, not because they exercise because they are healthy.

"Without the issues that are typically brought on by inactivity, their bodies have been permitted to age appropriately. If the activities were to stop, their health would probably go worse.

Both Dr. Ross Pollock, who conducted the muscle study, and Norman Lazarus, an emeritus professor at King's College London and an accomplished cyclist, concurred that: "Most of us who exercise have nowhere near the physiological capacity of great athletes.

"We work out primarily for enjoyment. Almost everyone can participate in an activity that is within their range of physiological ability.

"Find a form of exercise that you like to do in a setting that works for you, and establish regular physical activity. You'll benefit in the future by living an independent and fulfilling elderly age.

The Aging Antidotes.

Having Enough Sleep And Rest (Sleeping and Resting Enough.)

Perhaps just as crucial to aging health as food and exercise is sleep. Numerous studies have demonstrated that excessive or insufficient sleep is linked to death in older persons.

Numerous illnesses and chronic diseases, such as diabetes, cardiovascular disease, obesity, and depression, may all be made more likely by not getting enough sleep, according to a growing body of research.

This issue of PRB's Today's Research on Aging examines studies on sleep and aging that have received funding from the National Institute on Aging. It reviews fresh data suggesting that sleep deprivation may both be a sign of poor health and a catalyst for processes connected to disease and biological aging.

Even while it is common for older adults to have more difficulty getting and staying asleep, insomnia is not a given with aging. The studies reviewed here emphasize the significance of screening for poor sleep and sleep therapies for older persons.

The Aging Antidotes.

Sleepiness and Biological Aging.

Researchers are examining sleep's relationship to aging and chronic disease in greater detail. The majority of research on the connection between sleep length and health has relied on self-reported sleep duration. These studies show a U-shaped association between the amount of time spent sleeping and Mortality: The risk of mortality increases when people regularly sleep fewer than five hours per day or more than nine hours. 1

A more complex picture is provided by the examination of electronic sleep evaluation data that was amassed over several nights utilizing wristbands (actigraphy). According to research by the University of Chicago professor Diane Lauderdale and colleagues, sleeping fewer than six hours a night is connected to older adults having poor or fair health, whereas sleeping longer than average is not associated with any detrimental health effects. 2 More than 700 participants aged 62 to 90 who were included in the nationally representative National Social Life, Health, and Aging Project provided sleep data for their study (NSHAP). Our knowledge of how sleep affects health "may change as actigraphy matures," they write. One night of partial sleep

The Aging Antidotes.

deprivation activates genes linked to biological aging in older individuals, according to research from the University of California, Los Angeles. 29 senior citizens between the ages of 61 and 86 spent four nights in a sleep lab for the study. Participants were woken at 7 a.m. after two nights of unbroken sleep and were then prohibited from sleeping between the hours of 11 p.m. and 3 a.m. Daily blood samples were taken and sleep patterns were examined.

Participants' blood displayed symptoms of impairment in the cycle of cell growth and division following a night of partial sleep deprivation. According to the study's results, "sleep deprivation is causally linked to the molecular processes involved with biological aging," implying that lack of sleep may raise the risk of chronic disease by "activating the molecular pathways that drive biological aging."

By examining the findings from 72 different studies, Michael Irwin, Richard Olmstead, and Judith Carroll of the University of California, Los Angeles, discover more proof of the impact of sleep on the aging process. This body of work suggests that sleep disturbances (poor sleep or insomnia complaints) and long sleep

The Aging Antidotes.

duration (sleeping more than eight hours regularly) are related to increases in blood markers of inflammation. This body of work involved 50,000 participants in both clinical settings and the general population.

C-reactive protein (CRP) and interleukin-6, which are inflammatory indicators, are specifically linked to sleep disruption and excessive sleep (IL-6). These biomarkers frequently have connections to long-term diseases including diabetes and cardiovascular disease. Prior studies have demonstrated that treating insomnia can lower inflammation. In addition to high-fat diets and sedentary lifestyles, the researchers contend that sleep disruption and prolonged sleep length should be seen as additional risk factors for inflammation that may be altered. The fact that insomnia therapies may lower inflammatory indicators, for instance, provides proof that sleep issues might contribute to inflammation.

Depression and Sleep Issues Frequently Correspond.

Numerous studies have linked sleep deprivation with aging-related sadness.

Regardless of how many chronic medical illnesses a person has, a University of Michigan research found

The Aging Antidotes.

that poor sleep is linked to despair. The study followed more than 3,500 older persons who took part five times over a 25-year period in the nationally representative Americans' Changing Lives Study.

According to the study, depressed symptoms are more prevalent among older persons who have a larger number of chronic medical illnesses, such as high blood pressure, diabetes, chronic lung disease, heart attack or other cardiac problems, stroke, cancer, and arthritis. Poor sleepers who also have cardiac issues are at a higher risk of developing depressive symptoms.

According to the researchers, identifying sleep issues early and taking action to treat them with medication or behavioral modification can have long-term positive effects on both physical and mental health. Since those who suffer from depression often utilize more medical services than the average person, they make the case that early detection and treatment of sleep disorders might save costs and provide "enduring public health advantages."

Sleep disturbances that are really severe might indicate dementia.

The Aging Antidotes.

According to a group of Canadian experts, very disrupted sleep may be an early symptom of imminent dementia.

Prior to exhibiting other dementia-related symptoms, such as memory loss, elderly persons who are otherwise healthy may have disrupted sleep, including severe insomnia and daytime drowsiness. In order to conduct the study, the researchers looked at data gathered from more than 28,000 persons 50 and older who participated in the Survey of Health, Ageing, and Retirement (SHARE) in 12 different European nations.

Researchers developed a sleep disruption score using information from individuals who did not have any signs of Alzheimer's disease or dementia at the start of the trial (based on measures of sleep problems, fatigue, use of sleep medication, trouble sleeping, and changes in sleep patterns). According to analysis, each sleep metric is individually linked to a higher chance of developing Alzheimer's disease, dementia or passing away within four years. High scores on the sleep disruption index continue to be linked to a higher risk of dementia even after taking into account general health.

The Aging Antidotes.

People with dementia are known to have severe disruptions in their sleep-wake cycles and become quite active at night, placing a load on their family carers. In order to identify dementia early and begin therapies that may postpone or avoid institutionalization, the researchers advise healthcare professionals to screen for sleep issues in elderly patients.

The University of California, Berkeley study demonstrates that Alzheimer's-related sleep disturbances may differ from or be much worse than ordinary age-related sleep impairment.

A potentially non-invasive technique to detect persons at risk for Alzheimer's disease is to assess elderly adults for sleep abnormalities connected to the condition, such as reductions in non-rapid eye movement sleep. They contend that sleep deprivation is both "a result of the development of Alzheimer's disease and a cause of it; one that is adjustable, presenting promise for both preventive and therapeutic treatment."

According to a study conducted by scientists from California, Pennsylvania, Alabama, Maryland, and Illinois, regular sleep patterns of less than six hours

The Aging Antidotes.

each night may be associated with dementia-related brain abnormalities that can start as early as middle life.

In the Coronary Artery Risk Development in Young People (CARDIA) research, over 600 black and white adults (mean age 45) reported how long they typically slept before having brain MRIs five years later. Short sleepers' brains included more white matter hyperintensities (hardening of the brain's arteries) than individuals who slept between six and eight hours per night, which has been related to stroke and vascular dementia.

Affection And Sex(Touch and sex.)

How Sexual Behavior Alters with Age

The majority of people think that a person's sexual life naturally declines as they become older.

It is true that as people age, their bodies and minds change in ways that may have an impact on their sexuality.

This is not to say that sex needs to be "over" at a specific age or time. However, it does imply that some modifications frequently need to be taken into account in order to satisfy one's shifting requirements and physique.

Let's examine the typical aging-related changes that impact both men's and women's sex life.

"Intimacy sometimes leads to sex among men; sex sometimes leads to intimacy among women." Barb Cartland

How elderly women's sex differs

There is little question that a woman's sexual function alters as she ages, with sexual activity declining from 40% in women aged 65 to 74 to under 20% in those aged 75 to 85. If a male partner is less healthy or accessible, the fall in sexual activity may be accelerated since many elderly women define sex as vaginal intercourse. The more physically fit a woman is, the more likely she is to participate in sexual activity, and while her desire for closeness may wane, her need for sex does not.

The Aging Antidotes.

What alters:

Females who have gone through menopause have alterations to their sexual organs, which might provide difficulties:

Thickening and shrinking of the vulva and vaginal walls (Vulvovaginal atrophy)

less lubrication of the tissues around and within the vagina

higher sensitivity

Need for a longer arousal period

Therefore, for women:

Sexual activity may be painful.

Touch may be uncomfortable or grating.

Being prepared for sex frequently requires more time.

An orgasm might be postponed.

Steps to take:

To be evaluated for common medical disorders that may be causing or exacerbating their symptoms, women who

The Aging Antidotes.

are experiencing decreased libido or discomfort during sex should bring this up with their doctor.

And since the "Three T" basic intimacy tactics are excellent for assisting with these typical age-related changes impacting sexuality, it's nearly always a good idea to adopt (or review) one of them:

More time, more touch, and more talking

According to Natalie Wilton, timing is everything. "A lot of older women say their head feels turned on, but their body's not quite there yet," she says, adding that with a protracted arousal cycle, it might take up to 24 hours of "foreplay" to get physically ready.

A good experience might not require 24 hours of intense physical activity, but rather a long period of romance, tenderness, and connection. Talking during foreplay is permissible, but "More Talking" also refers to discussing the best ways to make sex more pleasant with your partner. This might involve purchasing a sex toy (online buying may be more convenient than visiting a physical store) and lubrication (readily available at most drug stores).

The Aging Antidotes.

Medication, such as topical (cream or vaginal suppository) or systemic (oral) hormone treatment, may be beneficial for certain women (usually only if there are other symptoms of menopause such as hot flashes, due to risks and side effects).

Last but not least, it's critical for women and their partners to understand how mental and interpersonal conditions might affect a woman's sexuality. After all, the sexual activity includes both the intellect and the body.

According to Natalie Wilton, the brain is the most significant sexual organ. Age-related health changes in their partner's body are one of the major influencers on older females' sexual desire and activity, according to Wilton. "It becomes thinking about sex in a new manner and doing things differently," he adds.

For many women, this entails changing the notion that having sex exclusively through vaginal contact is acceptable, experimenting with other sexual activities, and maybe even utilizing toys or other gadgets to enhance their sexual encounters with their partners.

The Aging Antidotes.

How elderly men's sex differs

Men seem to hold onto their desire and interest longer than women do as they age; up to 70% of people over the age of 70 reports engaging in sexual activity, with "real sex" often being described as penetrative penis-vagina contact.

What alters: Just as with women, older men may take longer to arouse and may want more time to pass after an orgasm before they are ready to start a new sexual cycle. Up to two-thirds of males over the age of 70 reports having erectile dysfunction, which is more prevalent as people get older.

This is frequently impacted by a variety of aging-associated illnesses and the drugs used to treat them, in addition to being tied to diminishing testosterone levels.

What to do: Since drugs are frequently the root of or a contributing factor in sexual problems, it is a good idea to discuss this with your doctor.

The Aging Antidotes.

The following is a list of the most popular drugs for erectile dysfunction to be aware of, categorized by the condition for which they are prescribed:

Medication for high blood pressure: beta-blockers, spironolactone, and thiazide diuretics

Opiates, a class of painkillers (e.g. Morphine, Hydromorphone)

Medication for enlarged prostate: 5 alpha-reductase inhibitors (e.g. finasteride)

Anti-androgens and other "testosterone blockers" are drugs used to treat prostate cancer.

Histamine-2 blockers as a treatment for stomach ulcers (e.g. ranitidine)

Tricyclic antidepressants, selective serotonin reuptake inhibitors, benzodiazepines, antipsychotics, and phenytoin are among the drugs for depression, anxiety, and other mood disorders.

Digoxin is a medicine for atrial fibrillation.

It is typically helpful for older men to reconsider their attitude to sex and intimacy, in addition to medication changes and treatment of other physical health issues.

The Aging Antidotes.

Reframing sex, for example, to place greater emphasis on sexual activities that don't require an erection or ejaculation, is a productive strategy when age or health issues lead to physical changes that are impossible to reverse. Older males value intimacy because they are more likely to be in a committed relationship than their mature female counterparts.

Despite getting older, many aspects of sex remain the same, particularly the emotional aspects, according to Natalie Wilton. Older folks may need to experiment with new methods and equipment to maintain a pleasant sexual life. Toys, lubricants, visual aids, or even a visit to a sex therapist are some examples of these.

Preventing Sex Abuse

At a later age, preventing pregnancy is typically not a concern. However, whether your partner is new or if you are unsure whether the relationship is exclusive, it is still necessary to wear condoms and engage in other safe sexual practices.

This is because older persons can and do have sexually transmitted diseases (STDs). Older people are less likely than younger people to get an STD, although the danger still exists. In reality, the following circumstances call for screening older women for STDs, according to the Centers for Disease Control:

New Companion

several sexual partners

Sex partners with partners who are also present

STD-carrying sex partner

Sex and Disability: Beyond Normal Aging

Some physical changes are universally accepted as normal, but what happens when sex is hampered by unforeseen health issues as people age? Instead of putting an end to a fulfilling sex life, in this section we'll discuss strategies for coping with problems that may come with aging.

Why bother?

If you're dealing with a handicap or condition, why even have sex? It benefits both your physical and mental well-being. For illustration:

Norepinephrine, serotonin, oxytocin, vasopressin, nitric oxide (NO), the hormone prolactin, and even

The Aging Antidotes.

endocannabinoid (your body's cannabis molecule) can all be released during sexual activity.

It increases confidence.

It encourages connection and intimacy.

It promotes the preservation of your sexual organs' health.

Strategies to help with common health concerns Caregivers who have happy sexual lives are happier than those who don't.

Pain:

Numerous illnesses, such as osteoarthritis, past traumas, neuropathic pain, or various stroke syndromes, include pain as a symptom. Making time for sex and intimacy in the middle of the day may be more joyful because many pain syndromes are more active in the morning or evening, which are traditional periods for sexual activity.

Natalie Wilton advises adjusting pillows or looking into acquiring specific foam wedges that might make sex more pleasant because positioning is crucial for those who live with pain.

The Aging Antidotes.

Cancer: After a cancer diagnosis, sex might alter significantly depending on the disease type and treatment approach. Sexual pleasure feelings and climax may not be experienced in the same physical manner as before. Sex may also be unable to continue. While receiving cancer treatment, some people lose interest in sex, but the majority desire to maintain or restart some form of sexual engagement, especially if they are in a committed relationship.

Many cancer treatment facilities have a social worker on staff who may offer assistance with the communication techniques required to renegotiate romantic relationships in the event of death or the loss of a bodily part due to disease. Practically speaking, mechanical devices and/or drugs can help with erectile function (like a vacuum or suction device).

Heart disease: Following a heart attack, significant cardiac procedure, or surgery, there may be a dread of having sex, similar to the fear experienced during cancer treatment. In general, when a person is well enough for exercise, they are also healthy enough for robust sexual activity, thus when recuperating from a heart attack or surgery, it may be necessary to explore

The Aging Antidotes.

activities like massage, hugging, or exchanging sexual dreams.

Many heart drugs can impair a man's ability to develop an erection and both a man and a woman's ability to experience orgasm, but quitting the prescription owing to these side effects might worsen symptoms and increase the chance of recurring episodes.

Parkinson's disease: The autonomic nervous system, which is involved in erections and orgasms, might experience rigidity, slowness, and other symptoms of Parkinson's. Scheduling sex at a medication's optimal efficacy can be crucial because many Parkinson's therapies have a predictable pattern of action.

Depression: Both mood disorders and the drugs used to treat them can have an impact on a person's libido and sexual performance. For instance, serotonin reuptake inhibitors, a frequently used antidepressant, might cause delayed arousal and make it more difficult to have an orgasm.

Dementia: Sex with a changing brain is sometimes presented as a problem or as "inappropriate," which might cause a person with dementia to take unneeded

The Aging Antidotes.

medications or isolate themselves from others. According to the World Health Organization, everyone has the right to sexual expression as long as it's safe and respectful, which is possible even when a person has dementia.

As you can see from the aforementioned examples, sex and health-related concerns are widespread and may be handled in a variety of ways. "Taking sexual activity off the table might be a place to start for many couples," says Wilton. Focusing on intimacy, pleasure, and emotional closeness rather than penis-vagina contact and orgasm can relieve strain and strengthen the bond between lovers.

When to consult a sex counselor

Professionals with specialized training in sex therapy include sex therapists, who may have backgrounds in social work, psychology, nursing, or medicine. Most deal with singles, and couples, and give counseling and advice.

Therapy entails: investigating the origins of difficulties

and instruction on useful tactics (e.g. positioning, use of aids)

The Aging Antidotes.

Using cognitive behavioral therapy, you may alter your ideas and habits. Even though those services may be offered by other experts, sex therapists usually never engage in sex surrogacy or have any physical contact with their clients.

Although some therapists focus on treating elderly people, many of the concerns that arise are universal and might include:

Incompatibility of the couples' levels of interest

Recovering From Adultery.

Managing the sexual aspect of a caring relationship and ensuring both partners' contentment with it

problems with female sexual health uncomfortable sexual encounters, issues with desire, climax

difficulties with male sexual health Erectile dysfunction delayed or early ejaculation

resuming sexual activity following a disease or injury

The conclusion

The Aging Antidotes.

The following are the main points that I want every senior (as well as every health professional!) to understand:

Throughout life, sexual activity is natural and crucial.

Male and female changes brought on by age may have an impact on sexual function and interest. Age-related health conditions might have an impact on sexual desire and performance.

Reorienting one's sexuality in later life may entail prioritizing sexual acts other than orgasm and penetration.

Strategies to enhance sexual health in older individuals include sex therapy, medication evaluation, and conversation with one's spouse. I hope this knowledge will motivate you to act and unlock the potential of your late-life sexual self if you have ever felt unsatisfied with your sex life or that you are "too old for this."

The Aging Antidotes.

Chapter 6
The Benefits of Aging.

The majority of senior citizens want to stay in their homes for as long as possible, even if others may feel better at ease with the amount of help provided by senior housing. Nearly 90% of seniors over 65 desire to age in place in their present residences, according to the AARP.

Independence is maintained

Maintaining one's sense of independence helps many people live a better quality of life as they age. As they may keep living in their familiar surroundings, older persons who age in place are able to maintain a high level of control over their life. People who are used to buying clothing, toiletries, and other requirements in their local communities sometimes find comfort in being able to handle these basics on their own. Their quality of life may increase if they feel sure that they can carry on without constant support.

To manage these everyday demands, older persons who are considering living with family or in senior living homes may need to ask for assistance or transportation. Why so many senior citizens opt to age in place may be due to a desire to preserve this feature of independence.

Some senior citizens place a lot of significance on maintaining tight ties to their assets. People who have spent years collecting items with significant significance, either financially or emotionally, may not like the idea of getting rid of them or even just rearranging them. Aging in place frequently allows older persons to continue enjoying their favorite activities on their terms, which may increase independence and satisfaction.

The Upkeep of Community Links

Aging in situ enables many senior citizens to carry on with their daily lives in much the same way that they have for many years. According to The New York Times, many older folks feel a great need to be connected to their neighborhoods and friends, with whom they may lose touch if they moved.

Older individuals can make social contact a regular part of their life by continuing to dwell in their communities. Maintaining vital friendships and vibrant social life can help older persons avoid dementia, which can lead to greater health and a higher standard of living.

Senior living communities may also provide a wealth of chances to form relationships and expand one's social network. However, moving forces senior citizens to form new acquaintances and could sever them from long-standing groups.

Budgeting Balance

For older persons who live on fixed monthly incomes, budgeting for the costs of healthcare, housing, support, and other essentials may not be simple. For some people, it might be difficult or even impossible to calculate the cost of moving into a senior living home.

Aging in place allows many older persons to have fewer monthly expenses and smaller housing budgets. About 20 percent of persons over 65 in the United States own their houses, according to the U.S. Department of Housing and Urban Development, and are thus exempt from including mortgage payments in their monthly budgets. Others could be qualified for the Federal Housing Administration's Home Equity Conversion

The Aging Antidotes.

Mortgage program, increasing the likelihood that many senior citizens would be able to age in place.

Since some homes where older individuals may reside have one or more flights of stairs, restricted toilet access, small corridors, and countless other mobility risks, it's critical to evaluate the safety

of each residence and deal with any pressing concerns as soon as possible. Starting early could also make it easier for elderly people to save aside the right amount of money for house renovations.

Making Whole Communities Flexible

In certain regions of the nation, planners have changed entire neighborhoods to accommodate an elderly population. The New York Times discusses how the Aging Improvement Districts in New York City have extended traffic signals and installed street crossings for senior citizens.

The Archstone Foundation has supported aging-in-place efforts for more than 20 years, including a number of villages around California. These programs in New York, California, and other

The Aging Antidotes.

places seek to keep older individuals active in their communities while promoting independent living for as long as feasible.

Seeking Assistance

In order to make house improvements or carry out everyday duties, older persons who want to age in place can find that they require assistance. Those who have earned a Master of Aging Services Management degree may be in a position to give senior citizens crucial help like this, such as aid with organizing renovations, handling money, or finding in-home care providers.

Additionally, gerontology experts may be able to assist senior citizens with difficulties like transportation, healthy eating, and even safety concerns. Geriatric care managers have the skills and information required to create long-term care plans and enhance the quality of life for older persons, even though many older adults may rely on family or friends for help.

The Aging Antidotes.

Conclusion.

While aging is unavoidable and part of life, it may also be hastened or resisted with anti-aging techniques. Whatever approach is used, it should be focused on three things: the mind, the inside of the body, and the body's external appearance. A minimum of twice every day, the skin must be washed, toned, and moisturized. Once every two weeks, a scrub gel is advised. As one provides a balanced diet to regulate weight, smoking and direct sunlight should also be avoided.

Regular exercise, whether it be a trip to the gym or just a simple stroll, should also be practiced, along with drinking plenty of water to aid with toxin removal and getting adequate sleep. Humans are urged to keep a positive outlook on the life events they are going through since stress has been shown to speed up aging. The diet should also include a lot of antioxidant vitamins, the majority of which may be found in locally accessible, natural fruits and vegetables. A person may also depend on synthetic antioxidants if natural ones are unavailable.

The Aging Antidotes.

According to the wear-and-tear idea, environmental harm to the body's systems accumulates over time and is the root cause of aging. Internal or external damage, which both result in "tear and wear" of the bodily cells, is what causes the damage. The body eventually dies as a consequence of these damage-related effects, including tissue and cell wear and tear. When biological molecules are harmed, the consequences build up over time, but the DNA, which is in charge of creating the genes, minimizes these effects.

However, the body may not be particularly good at completely getting rid of all these consequences. Chemicals used to tone the skin, some of which are abrasive and uncomfortable, as well as those used in laundry that react with the skin, are some of the ways that the tear and wear occur.

Molecules that are free radicals and have charges due to unbound electrons. The molecule may be destroyed by interacting with other very volatile compounds thanks to the electron. Although having an electrical charge imbalance to allow for chemical reactions is normally helpful for the body, it does have negative repercussions. In order to find an electron to pair with

The Aging Antidotes.

and achieve electrical equilibrium, the free radical joins forces with other molecules as a consequence of the imbalance. The body sustains significant harm as a result of the breakdown of the coupled electrons.

From birth till death, the effects of the free radical are felt. Since the body has a complex system in place to replace damaged cells, its impact is minimal in youth, but as we age, the consequences become more pronounced. Collagen and gelatin, which are important for moisturizing and smoothing the skin and keeping it elastic and supple, may also be damaged by free radicals. Free radical damage over time causes the soft tissues to shred, resulting in folds and deep cut creases, notably on the face.

By protecting the skin from the sun with specific lotions like SPF 15, a large portion of wrinkles that develop on a person's skin may be prevented. Sunglasses are also advised because they stop direct UV radiation from entering the eyes, which causes individuals to squint repeatedly. The squinting is what has the most impact on the development of wrinkles around the eyes. A second habit that many people are unaware of is holding the cheek with one or both hands when sitting

The Aging Antidotes.

or even standing, as well as wrinkling the brow since these actions can generate cheek wrinkles. It is recommended that people use the appropriate facial expressions throughout their whole lifespan.

Smoking is not recommended for healthy skin, and if it is necessary, smoking should be done very seldom since it may lead to lines around the lips from repeated mouth openings. The quantity of oxygen accessible for the skin is further decreased by the harmful chemicals included in cigarettes, such as carbon (II) oxide. Balms and eye shadows are excellent moisturizers since they make the skin and face seem nice when they are soft. Several food irritants that are known to aggravate inflammation. When the body is invaded or in the presence of an irritant, inflammation is the body's response. It is recommended that a person eat less or no irritants like sugar in their diet, only healthy fats, and get enough sleep. Alcohol should only be used in moderation since it includes harmful chemicals that lead to the production of free radicals. Although red wine itself is an antioxidant, it is advised to drink it in moderation since there is no evidence to support the notion that the advantages outweigh the drawbacks.

The Aging Antidotes.

High temperatures during food preparation may cause the fat to break down and release free radicals, particularly when nuts are roasted for commercial purposes and certain oils that are heat sensitive break down and produce radicals. This is particularly typical in grilled meat, where it may be reduced by slow cooking and putting rosemary, an antioxidant, to the meat before grilling to combat free radicals brought on by high temperatures.

The Aging Antidotes.